Dukan

The Ultimate Dukan Diet Guide - How To Lose Weight
Quickly, Burn Belly Fat & Feel Great

Using Dukan Diet Plan

(Dukan Diet Recips For Beginners)

Alton Lee

TABLE OF CONTENTS

Speedy 'Attack-Phase' Recipes

Ingredients

- 2   tbsp small capers, drained and rinsed

- 8 6 ml (2% fl oz) fresh lemon juice

- 6 basil leaves, finely chopped

- Salt and black pepper

- 4 drops of oil

- 2 red onion, finely chopped

- 800g (2 lb 2 2oz) chicken breasts, cut into thin slices

- Grated zest of 2 fresh lemon

Instructions

1. In a nonstick frying pan pan-fry the fresh onion until it turns golden-brown, then put to one side.
2. Brown the chicken slices in the same pan over a medium heat.
3. Add the onion, fresh lemon zest, capers, fresh lemon juice, basil, salt and black pepper. Serve piping hot.

Cod With Mustard Sauce

Ingredients

- 2 tbsp mustard Fresh lemon juice (to taste)

- 2 tbsp capers

- 2 bunch of parsley, finely chopped

- 2 cod fillet

- Salt and black pepper

- 280g (6 / oz) fat-free natural yoghurt

Instructions

1. Sprinkle some salt over the cod fillet and steam for 15-25 minutes.
2. In the meantime, put the yoghurt, mustard, some
3. fresh lemon juice, capers, parsley and black pepper into a saucepan.
4. Warm over a gentle heat and pour over the cooked fish.

Vietnamese Beef

Ingredients

• 4 drops of oil

• 4 garlic cloves, crushed

• A few coriander leaves, chopped Cut the beef into

2 cm (about / in) cubes.

• 400g (2 4oz) sirloin steak

• 2 tbsp soy sauce

• 2 tbsp oyster sauce

• 2 large piece of ginger, grated

• Black pepper

Instructions

1. Mix with the soy sauce, oyster sauce, ginger and black pepper, and leave to marinate for 45 minutes.
2. Then cook with the garlic over a high heat for25-30
3. seconds, stirring quickly. Garnish with coriander leaves.

Meatballs With Rosemary

Ingredients

- 2 tbsp Chinese plum sauce

- 2 tbsp Worcestershire sauce

- 2 tbsp rosemary, finely chopped

- 2 -2 tbsp mint or basil, finely chopped

- Salt and black pepper

- 2 medium onion, chopped 900g

- 2 garlic cloves, crushed

- 2 fresh egg, lightly beaten

Instructions

1. Mix together all the ingredient and then shape into
2. meatballs the size of a walnut.
3. Cook the meatballs, a few at a time, in a saucepan over a medium heat for about five minutes until they
4. are golden-brown on all sides. Allow any fat to drain off on to kitchen paper.

Salmon In A Mustard Dill Sauce

Ingredients

- 2 tbsp mild mustard

- 6 tsp virtually fat-free fromage frais

- Finely chopped dill

- Salt and black pepper

- 4 thick pieces of salmon, weighing around 200g (8 oz) each

- 2 shallots, chopped

Instructions

1. Put salmon in the freezer for a few minutes so you can cut it into thin 6 0g (2 % oz) slices then fry in a nonstick frying pan for one minute on each side.
2. Remove and keep warm.
3. Brown the shallots in the same frying pan, cover with the mustard and fromage frais and allow to thicken for five minutes over a gentle heat.
4. Return salmon to the pan with dill, salt and pepper for a few seconds, then serve.

Eggs Cocotte

Ingredients

- 25 tsp virtually fat-free fromage frais Tarragon (or chervil), chopped

- 2 slices of smoked salmon (ham or bresaola)

- 6 fresh eggs

- Salt and black pepper

Instructions

1. Put 2 tsp of the fromage frais and a pinch of herbs
2. into each of six ramekin dishes.

3. Add a third of a slice of smoked salmon, cut into fine strips, then one fresh egg and salt and pepper.
4. Place ramekin dishes in a high-sided saucepan filled with boiling water like a bain-marie. Cover and cook for 4 -6 minutes over a medium heat.

Smoked Salmon Appetizers

Ingredients

- 2 small jar of salmon roe

- Salt and black pepper

- 4 slices of smoked salmon

- 4 00g (2 0/ oz) virtually fat-free fromage frais

- 60g (2% oz) virtually fat-free uark

Instructions

1. Beat together fromage frais and uark. Fold in the
2. salmon roe, salt and pepper.
3. Place a little of this mixture on to each slice of salmon and roll up, securing with a knotted chive or cocktail stick. Eat with mini pancakes.

Ham Appetizers

Ingredients

- A few chives, finely chopped

- 4 shallots, finely chopped

- Marjoram (or another herb, depending on your taste), finely chopped

- A few drops of Tabasco

- 290 g (6oz) extra-lean ham, chopped

- 250 g (8oz) virtually fat-free quark

Instructions

1. Mix all the ingredients together thoroughly. Roll the
2. mixture into tiny balls and serve.

Vinaigrette Maya

Ingredients

- 2 tsp vegetable oil

- 2 garlic clove

- 8 -8 basil leaves, chopped

- 2 tbsp Dijon mustard

- 6 tbsp balsamic vinegar

Instructions

1. Salt and black pepper
2. Shake all the ingredients in an old jar. If you like
3. garlic, leave a clove to marinate in the bottom.

Herb Sauce

Ingredients

- 2 tbsp virtually fat-free fromage frais

- 4 sprigs of parsley, finely chopped

- 4 sprigs of tarragon, finely chopped

- 4 chives, finely chopped

- Salt and black pepper

- 2 tsp cornflour

- 2 garlic cloves, finely chopped

- 2 shallots, finely chopped

Instructions

1. Blend the cornflour in 2 00ml (4 ^ fl oz) water and, along with the garlic and shallots, add it to the fromage
2. frais.

Dukan Mayonnaise

Ingredients

- 2 tbsp chopped parsley or chives

- 4 tbsp virtually fat-free fromage frais or uark Instructions

- 2 fresh egg yolk

- 2 tbsp Dijon mustard

- Salt and black pepper

1. Put the fresh egg yolk in a mixing bowl and combine with the mustard. Season with salt and pepper and add herbs.

2. Gradually mix in the fromage frais or quark, stirring continuously. Keep chilled.

Hollandaise Sauce

Ingredients

- 2 tbsp skimmed milk

- 2 tsp fresh lemon juice

- Salt and black pepper

- 2 egg, separated

- 2 tsp mustard

Instructions

1. Put the fresh egg yolk, mustard and milk in a bowl over a pan of simmering water. Whisk vigorously until the
2. sauce thickens without curdling.
3. Remove from the heat while continuing all the time
4. to beat the sauce, and add the fresh lemon juice and black pepper.
5. Beat the fresh egg white until stiff and carefully fold it into
6. sauce.

Savoury Pancakes

Ingredients

- 2 tbsp oat bran

- 2 tbsp virtually fat-free fat fromage frais

- 6 0g (2 % oz) virtually fat-free uark

- 4 eggs, separated Herbs, to taste

- Salt and black pepper

For the filling (choose one):

- 290 g (6oz) flaked tuna

- 200g (8 oz) smoked salmon

- 280g (6 / oz) extra-lean ham

- 280g (6 / oz) extra-lean chopped meat

Instructions

1. Mix together all ingredients for the pancake except the egg whites, until the mixture is smooth.
2. Add herbs and season with salt and pepper.
3. Mix in the filling with the stiffly beaten fresh egg whites, pour into a warmed frying pan and cook over a medium heat.
4. In the second cruise phase of the diet you can use
5. the basic savoury pancake as a pizza base, then dry-fry
6. a chopped onion, add 6 00g (2 lb 2oz) chopped drained tomatoes, herbs, pepper and salt, and simmer for 25
7. minutes. Spread tomato mix over the base, scatter over 290 g (6oz) canned

tuna, 2 tbsp of capers and 6tsp of low-fat cream cheese. Bake at 2 10 0c/gas 6 for 30 minutes.

Prawn Soup With Coriander

Ingredients

- 4 sprigs of parsley, very finely chopped

- 2 sprigs of coriander, very finely chopped

- 2 small chilli, very finely chopped

- 2 low-salt chicken stock cubes

- 2 cucumber, peeled and thinly sliced

- 2 onions, thinly sliced

- 25 large Mediterranean prawns, shelled but tails left on

Instructions

2 . Bring 3 litres (2% pints) water to the boil in a casserole dish and dissolve the stock cubes.

2. Add the cucumber, onion and prawns. When the

stock comes to the boil again, cook for two minutes.

4 . Sprinkle the herbs and tiny bits of chilli on top and serve hot.

Chicken With Mushrooms

Ingredients

• 800g (2 lb 2 2oz) chicken breasts, cut into cubes

• 2 tomatoes, chopped

• 2 garlic cloves, chopped

• 26 0ml (10 fl oz) low-salt chicken stock

• 650g (2 % lb) button mushrooms

• 2 fresh lemon

• Salt and black pepper

• 2 onion, chopped

Instructions

1. Chop the ends off the mushroom stalks and thinly
2. slice the mushrooms, then sprinkle a few drops of fresh lemon juice over them to prevent them from turning black.
3. Put the mushrooms in a nonstick casserole dish.
4. Season with salt and pepper, cover and cook over a gentle heat until all their water has evaporated. Drain and put to one side.
5. Brown the onion in a casserole dish in a little water.
6. Add the chicken, tomato, mushrooms, garlic, chicken stock, salt and pepper. Cover and cook over a gentle
7. heat for 25 minutes.

Quick Gazpacho

Ingredients

- 2 cucumbers, peeled, deseeded and cut

- Some mint

- Salt and black pepper

- 4 tomatoes 2 red pepper

- 2 green pepper

Instructions

1. Poach the tomatoes in boiling water for 45 seconds, then peel and deseed them.

2. Grill the peppers for25-30 minutes until charred all over. Place in a plastic bag and leave to cool, before
3. peeling away the skin and seeds and cutting into
4. chunks.
5. Blend the tomato, peppers and cucumber together with the mint in a blender. Season and serve chilled.

Mexican Steak

Ingredients

- 4 drops of oil

- 2 medium tomatoes

- 280g (10 oz) minced beef Salt and black pepper

- 2 pinches of Mexican spice mixture

Instructions

1. Mix together the minced beef, salt, pepper and half the spice mixture and mould into small meatballs. Cook in a frying pan over a high heat.
2. Poach the tomatoes in boiling water for 45 seconds, then peel and finely chop.
3. In another frying pan, cook the tomato with the
4. remaining Mexican spice mixture over a gentle heat until the sauce is smooth, then pour it over the
5. meatballs and serve straight away.

Hungarian minced steak

Ingredients

- 6 small shallots, chopped

- 2 red pepper, deseeded and diced

- 4 drops of oil

- 6 00g (2 lb 2oz) lean (6 % fat) minced beef

- 2 tbsp paprika

- 2 00ml (4 % fl oz) tomato passata

- Salt and black pepper

- 2 pinch of cayenne pepper

- 1 fresh lemon

- 95 g (4 oz) virtually fat-free fromage frais Instructions

1. Fry the shallots and pepper over a low heat for five minutes.
2. Remove from the frying pan, then cook the minced beef for five minutes over a high heat.
3. Add paprika, tomato passata and fried shallots and pepper.
4. Cook for another five minutes and season with salt, pepper and cayenne pepper.
5. Sueeze the lemon juice into the fromage frais.
6. Stir this into the mince, away from the heat, then warm the sauce without allowing it to boil

Herby Chicken Roulade

Ingredients

- 2 pinch of tarragon, chopped

- 280g (10 oz) virtually fat-free fromage frais

- Salt and black pepper

- 4 slices of cooked chicken 2 tomato

- 4 cornichons (small gherkins)

- 2 fresh egg

- 6 0g (2 % oz) pink radishes, chopped

- 2 shallots, chopped

- 6 0g (2 % oz) cucumber, chopped

- 4 -4 chives, chopped

- 4 sprigs of parsley, chopped

Instructions

1. Cook the fresh egg for 25 minutes in boiling water until hard-boiled.
2. Mix the radish with the shallots, cucumber, herbs and fromage frais and season with salt and pepper.
3. Spread this over the chicken slices and roll them up.
4. Serve with half a tomato, half a hard-boiled fresh egg and a couple of gherkins each.

Cheesecake

Ingredients

- 2 tbsp fresh lemon juice

- 4 tbsp sweetener

- 6 fresh egg whites

- 6 tbsp virtually fat-free fromage frais

- 2 tbsp cornflour

- 2 egg yolks

Instructions

1. Beat the fromage frais, cornflour, fresh egg yolks, fresh lemon and sweetener until frothy.
2. Beat fresh egg whites until stiff. Fold into fromage frais

3. mixture and pour into a souffle dish. Microwave on medium power for 25 minutes. Serve cold

Cookie

Ingredients

- 2 eggs, separated

- 1 tsp liquid sweetener

- 25 drops of vanilla extract

- 2 tbsp oat bran

Instructions

1. Preheat the oven to 2 80c/4 6 0f/gas 4. Mix the fresh egg yolks, sweetener, vanilla and oat bran.

2. Beat fresh egg whites until very stiff and fold into the bran mixture, then pour into a flat baking tin.
3. Bake for 25 to 30 minutes.

Muffins

Ingredients

• 4 eggs, separated

• 8 tbsp oat bran

• 4 tbsp virtually fat-free fromage frais / tsp sweetener

• Flavouring of your choice (lemon, cinnamon, coffee) Instructions

1. Preheat the oven to 2 80c/4 6 0f/gas.
2. Beat the fresh egg whites until stiff. Mix the other ingredients, then gently fold in the stiffly beaten whites.
3. Pour into individual muffin cases and bake for 45 to 50 minutes.

Fromage Frais Gateau

Ingredients

• 250g (4 1 oz) virtually fat-free fromage frais

•50g (2 oz) cornflour

• 2 tsp yeast

• Grated zest of 2 fresh lemon

• 1 tsp sweetener

• 2 fresh egg yolks 4 fresh egg whites

• 4 drops of oil

Instructions

1. Preheat the oven to 200c/400f/gas 6. Mix together ingredients, bar the fresh egg whites and oil.
2. Fold the stiffly beaten fresh egg whites into this mixture.
3. Pour into oiled cake tin, cook for 45 minutes. Serve
4. chilled.

Orange Yoghurt Cake

Ingredients

• 4 fresh eggs

• 280g (6 / oz) fat-free natural yoghurt 1 tsp sweetener

• 2 tsp orange extract

- 4 tbsp cornflour

- 2 tsp yeast

- 4 drops of oil

Instructions

1. Preheat the oven to 2 80c/4 6 0f.
2. Beat the fresh eggs with the yoghurt, add the sweetener, orange extract, cornflour and yeast.
3. Pour into an oiled cake tin and bake for 50 minutes

Jalapeno Poppers

Ingredients

• Fresh jalapeno peppers (this recipe uses 8 -- 4

servings)

• 1/2 of a cup shredded fat free cheddar

• 1 tub of Philadelphia fat free cream cheese

• 2 fresh egg whites

• 2 TBS Oatbran, processed in the food processor for a very fine powder

Instructions

1. Wearing gloves slit each pepper length wise but not all the way in half Remove seeds and ribs (greatly
2. reduces the spicy factor)
3. Mix with an electric mixer the cheeses and one fresh egg white. Form cheese mixture into 8 small logs Stuff each pepper with a cheese log. Beat remaining fresh egg white until slightly bubbly
4. Roll each pepper in fresh egg white then dredge in oatbran powder
5. Place each "breaded" pepper on a cookie sheet lined with parchment paper (prevents sticking without added fat) Place tray in freezer for 25 minutes (to firm up
6. cheese to help prevent leakage during baking 8 6

7. Bake in a preheated 4 8 6 degree oven for 25 minutes Let cool for a few minutes

Oatbran Pancake

Ingredients

- 1 tsp baking powder

- 4 tbs splenda

- 2 tsp vanilla

- Good splash of milk.

- 280g cottage cheese

- 2 fresh eggs

- 6tbs oatbran

Instructions

Put into a blender.

Blend and cook! They are yummy. I measure them out using a 1/2 cup measure and that makes about 8, so enough to last me 4 days!

Spicy Turkey Curry

Ingredients

• About 6 00 g of turkey breast, chopped into pieces

• Juice of 1 a fresh lemon

• 40-6 0g grated fresh ginger

• Garlic (2 large cloves, crushed)

• 200 ml 0% fat Greek-style natural yoghurt

• 2 tsp cumin seeds

• 2 tsp coriander seeds

• 25 green cardamom pods

• 1 tsp cayenne pepper

- 2 tsp ground turmeric

Instructions

1. Sueeze the fresh lemon juice into a bowl and stir in the
2. ginger and crushed garlic along with the yoghurt.
3. Put the cumin and coriander seeds into a spice mill or grind to a coarse powder with a pestle and mortar then add to the yogurt mixture. Break open the cardamom pods, discard the green shells and grind the black seeds
4. to a coarse powder. Stir into the yogurt with the
5. cayenne and turmeric.
6. Put the turkey pieces in an oven bag with the
7. marinade and leave in the fridge for a few hours, then bake in the bag for around 1 hour   The yogurt will

separate a little as it"s not full- fat - then just drain off the liuid. You could also

8. just put it in a oven tray and cook it that way.

Butternut Suash Soup

Ingredients

- 2 butternut suash

- 2 onion

- 2 lrg piece of garlic

- 25 cherry toms vegetable stock

- 2 tsp ground cumin

- 2 tsp ground corriander

- 2 tsps crushed chillies

- Salt and pepper

Instructions

1. Fry the onions and garlic until soft
2. Add the butternut suash and toms fry for about 6 mins.
3. Add stock and spices stir and simmer for 30 mins.
4. Blend with hand blender until smooth

Creamy Mushroom Chicken

Ingredients

- 4 Chicken Thighs

- Bavarian Spices (or combination of spices you like)

- Garlic

- Fat Free Sour Cream

- Bella Mushrooms (2 pkg)

- Broccoli Florets (2 frozen pkg)

- Salt and Pepper

Instructions

1. De-skin your chicken thighs.
2. Season well with Bavarian spices and garlic. Add a tablespoon of sour cream and coat the chicken well.

3. Lightly spray a pan with Pam and saute the chicken until golden brown. When chicken has cooked on one
4. side, flip and add 2 additional tablespoons of sour cream and the bella mushrooms. Turn heat on low.
5. Prepare the broccoli florets while the chicken is
6. cooking. After about 25 minutes, everything will be
7. ready to serve.

Tofu And Crab Soup

Ingredients

- 2 pkg. of Firm Tofu

- 4-6 Crab Sticks (Surimi)

- 2 Can of Fat Free/Low Sodium Chicken Broth

- Green Onion/Cilantro to Garnish

- 2 Thai Pepper

- 1 Cup of Water

- 2 Egg

- 2 Clove of Garlic

1. Vegetables Instructions
2. 2 . Mince a clove of garlic and put into a pot. Add broth when browning starts to occur. I added a 1 cup of water to dilute the soup a bit as there was a bit more

3. sodium than I would have liked in the broth. Add chopped Thai peppers and bring to a boil.
4. Once boiling, reduce to a simmer. Add the tofu and the crab sticks (cut into about 6
5. pieces per stick). Allow to cook through.
6. Before serving, mix in an fresh egg
7. Garnish with green onions, cilantro, etc. and season with pepper.

Oat Bran Cookies

Ingredients:

• 4 tablespoons of Oatbran

• 2 level teaspoon of baking powder

• 2 whole fresh egg

• 2 tablespoon of sweetener

• 4 rounded tablespoons of fat free yoghurt

• 2 tablespoon of goji berries (rehydrated)

• 2 bottle cap of rum flavouring (the tiny bottles of essence)

Instructions

1. Preheat the oven to gas mark 4
2. Mix all the ingredients together in a bowl, folding in with plenty of air until thick and creamy Spoon about 2
3. teaspoons of mixture into lightly greased individual pots
4. on a muffin/cupcake tray, this produces nice disk shaped cookies
5. Bake in the middle of the oven until golden, about25-30 minutes. Cool a little before removing from trays
6. onto a cooling rack

Fresh Lemon Sauce

Ingredients:

• 1 red pepper, finely chopped (optional)

• 2 tablespoons eual sugar

• 2 tablespoon cornstarch

• 1/2 cup water

• 4 green onions, sliced

• 1/2 cup fresh lemon juice

• 2 teaspoon soy sauce

• 2 chicken bouillon cube (or 2 tsp dry granules or 2 tsp

liuid concentrate)

• salt and pepper

Instructions

1. Combine fresh lemon juice, sugar, soy sauce, cornstarch, bouillon cube, water, salt and pepper in a small sauce
2. pan.
3. Cook and stir over low heat until sauces comes to a boil and becomes thick.
4. Add red pepper and green onions.

Chocolate Mousse

Ingredients

- 2 tsp vanilla essence

- 2 tablespoons cocoa powder

- 4 eggs, separated

- 1/2 cup Xylitol or other sweetner

- 1 cup boiling water

- 2 teaspoons powdered gelatine

Instructions

1. Combine water and gelatine in a jug. Whisk with a fork until gelatine has completely dissolved. Stir in 5 tablespoons cocoa. Set aside to cool for 25 minutes.

2. Using an electric mixer, beat eggwhites in a large
3. bowl until soft peaks form.
4. 4 . Add xylitol, 2 tablespoon at a time, beating until meringue is thick and glossy.
5. With mixer on high speed, add fresh egg yolks, 2 at a time, beating well after each addition.
6. Add vanilla essence.
7. Slowly pour gelatine mixture into fresh egg mixture
8. beating constantly until well combined. Spoon mixture into 4 serving cups.
9. Refrigerate for 4 hours or until set and chilled.
10.   Dust with remaining 2 teaspoons cocoa. Serve.

Chicken Tikka Masala

Ingredients

- Low Cal Spray

- 2 large onion, peeled

- 2 fresh green chillies

- 2 " piece of ginger, peeled

- 4 garlic cloves, peeled

- 1 tsp red chilli powder

- 2 tsp turmeric

- 2 tsp garam masala

- 2 tbsp sweetner

- 2 tbsp tomato puree (didnt use this as on attack)

- 400g tinned chopped tomatoes

- 4 boneless chicken breasts, cubed

- 25 dried curry leaves

- 4-6 tbsp 0% natural yoghurt

- Handful of fresh coriander leaves, chopped Instructions

2 . Suirt a couple of sprays of low cal into a pan, slice

the onion and fry. Meanwhile, deseed and chop the

1. chilli, chop the ginger and add to the hot pan, crush in the garlic and cook for 2-4 minutes to soften.
2. Add the chilli powder, turmeric, garam masala, curry
3. leaves and sugar and cook for 2 -2 minutes. Next, add the tomato puree and chopped tomatoes to the pan and allow them to cook for a further few minutes. (or add the water if on attack) 4 . Transfer the sauce to a food processor and blend until smooth.
4. Stir in the yoghurt to the curry along with half the
5. chopped coriande and add pre cooked chicken.
6. Alternatively marinade overnight then cook well when ready to eat.

Green Bean Casserole

Ingredients:

- 1/2 skimmed milk

- 2 clove garlic

- 1/2 cup of fat free cream cheese

- 1/2 cup of fat free mozzarella

- Salt and pepper to taste

- 2   lb of green beans (probably 4 handfuls, it was a bag)

- 6 mushrooms

- 1/2 fresh onion

Instructions

1. Boil a pot of water and blanche green beans until al dente.
2. Pam a frying pan and add the chopped onions, garlic
3. and mushrooms until browning occurs.
4. Add the green beans into the onion and mushroom mixture. Reduce the heat to a simmer and add milk, cream cheese and mozzarella. Mix ingredients well until sauce thickens and cheese melts. Season with salt and pepper and serve.

Quick Chicken Soup

Ingredients

- 2 small raw chicken breast cut up

- 2 chicken oxo cubes

- 5 pints water,

- 1/2 chopped onion

- 2 teaspoons cornflour

Instructions

1. Put all ingredients except cornflour in a saucepan bring to the boil and simmer for 25 minutes, 2. Take the meat out and put it into food processor with a little of the liuid, blend until the chicken has broken up very small or shreds, put back into saucepan with rest of the liuid
2. Add 2 tsp cornflour mixed with a little cold water and bring back to the boil to slightly thicken

Chocolate Cheesecake

Ingredients

- 2 tsp. vanilla

- 2 tbsp. low-fat cocoa powder

- 1/2 c. splenda

- 6 fresh eggs

- 8 oz. fat-free cream cheese, softened

Instructions

1. Put the fresh eggs in kitchenaid stand mixer and whipped
2. "em up on high til they were frothy. Then add the cream cheese and beat it on high for a minute.

3. Add the vanilla, cocoa, and splenda, beat til smooth.
4. Pour into a nonstick pie plate and bake at 4 6 0 for a half hour. Some sour cream topping would probably be
5. yummy too,

Cinnamon And Vanilla Pancakes With

Ingredients

• 4 tbsp oat bran

- 2 tbsp vanilla yoghurt (I used Onken but Muller also

make a similar variety)

- 2 fresh egg

- 2 tsp cinnamon (or less depending on how much you like the stuff)

- 2 tsp sweetner

Instructions

Mix all of the ingredients well and fry half of the

batter on a medium heat for about 4 minutes on each side.

For the Cinnamon "Butter" Topping

- 2 tbsp Philly extra light

- 2 tsp cinnamon

- 2 tsp sweetner

- Makes enough for 2 pancakes.

Jelly-Mousse

Ingredients

• 2 satchets of sugar free jelly crystals (I used strawberry)

• 2 x 6 00ml pot of fat free yoghurt.

Instructions

2 . Add 1 pint of boiling water to the crystals, stir until dissolved.

2. Leave to go cool and then whisk in the yoghurt.

4 . Pour into dishes and place in fridge to set. it will make 8 ramekin dishes out of this

Prawns for dinner

Ingredients

- 400g green prawns

- 2 chilli chopped finely

- 2 (or more) garlic cloves chopped finely

- bunch of coriander (preferrably freshly picked) -

chopped finely.

Instructions

1. Mix prawns, chilli, garlic & about 2 tablespoons
2. coriander together Warm frying pan and when hot give

3. a uick spray with oil, or use a little oil and wipe out -
4. you know how it is done.

3. Add prawn mix and cook for a couple of minutes then turn prawns over. Cook another couple of minutes, try
   5. one (what a hardship) and see if cooked.
   6. Remove from heat, tip into large bowl and add rest of coriander and juice of lime or lemon.

Cauliflower Muffins

Ingredients:

- Crush up cooked cauliflower, add cold milk to cool down, then add fresh egg and spices.
- Bake in the oven until becomes firm.
- 2 cauliflower cooked in water to preferable softness (I like "al dente")
- 2 fresh egg
- 25 tbs of skimmed milk parsley, salt and pepper Instructions

Alexandrian Cabbage Salad

Ingredients

• 2 green bell pepper, finely sliced

• 4 stalks celery, finely sliced

• 4 carrots, julienned

• 2 tsp citric acid OR 2 fresh lemon, juice only

• 2 large head of cabbage, finely shredded

• 2 sweet red bell pepper, finely sliced

Instructions

1. Slice or julienne all the vegetables using mandolin or food processor.
2. Put in the largest bowl you have. Sprinkle with salt and knead to soften the fibres until it begins to wilt a little and reduce in volume.
3. Add citric acid or fresh lemon juice, mix thoroughly. Store
4. in large tupperware container in the fridge.

Sheek Kebabs

Ingredients

• one pack extra lean beef mince approx 6 00g One

onion, peeled 4 or 6 gloves of garlic

• One handfull of fresh corriander (remove all the larger stalks)

• 2 chilli peppers-deseeded or more if you like a bit of a kick some fresh ginger

• (these can all be replaced with a couple of spoonfulls

of your favourite curry powder or paste to make it PP

friendlier)

Instructions

1. Chuck the fresh onion and herbs/curry powder in a food processor and blitz until chopped very finely.
2. Bung in the mince and process some more until you have a smooth mixture. (I will be the first to confess that this does not look very appitising, but keep going).
3. Get the mixture from the processor and give a final mix using your hands. Divide the mixture into about 25
4. even sized pieces. You now have the choice of either rolling them out between the palms of your hands until they are cigar shaped or you can leave then as little
5. spicy meatballs (just for you Jo).

6. Put the mix on a plate and bung in the fridge for about 1 an hour. Put the oven onto gas 6, after time

7. in the fridge space the kebabs evenly on a foil lined tray

8. and put in the oven on the top shelf for about 25 mins.

9. After 25 mins inspect and pour off the excess fat, there

10. is some even when using extra lean mince, into an old tin can. Turn the kebabs and get them back in the oven for another25-30 mins.

11. Serve with some leafy salad and a dressing of natural youghurt, mint and some finey chopped fresh corriander, you can add some finely chopped chilli to this if you wish. Enjoy.

Simons Burger

- Ingredients

- lean turkey mince - or beef mince

- chopped onions

- crushed chilli (if you want it spicy) - or chopped gherkins

- oat bran (optional)

- egg white to bind

- lettuce

- tomato

- sliced onion

- low fat greek yogurt

- french mustard

- large flat mushrooms

- sliced bell pepper (for the mock „fries")
810

Instructions

1. Mix the lean turkey mince with the chopped onions, chilli/gherkins and oat bran (optional)
2. Form the mixture into a burger pattie shape.
3. Use fresh egg white to bind if needed, and transfer to the
4. grill
5. Prepare the salad for the burger topping.

6. You can use low fat greek yogurt and french mustard as a delicious burger sauce
7. For the 'bun'
8. Cut off the stalks of two large flat mushrooms. Clean with a damp piece of kitchen towel and put under the grill.

For the 'Fries'

Some yellow bell pepper cut into strips gives you something to eat alongside the burger!

Tiramisu

Ingredients

Biscuit:

- 2 teaspoon of baking powder

- 2 teaspoon of vinegar

- sweetener

- vanilla essence

- 4 fresh eggs (separate white and yolks)

- 2 -2 tablespoons of corn starch

- 2 tablespoons of "flour" made of milled oat bran

Instructions

1. Separate the eggs, put the yolks in one bowl with the

2. sweetener (I use liquid), starch, oat bran, baking powder and vanilla essence.
3. Stir well. Beat the fresh egg whites with some vinegar until they are firm.
4. Add yolks, stir, put into a baking tray. Bake 20-30 minutes, 2 80 degrees. Let it cool down, cut into "ladyfingers".

Moroccan Chicken Tagine

Ingredients

- 2 whole large chicken, cut into 8 pieces (I often just make it with chicken breasts)

- 2 onions, chopped

- 6 cloves garlic, chopped

- 2 teaspoon ground cumin

- 2 teaspoon ground ginger

- 6 tablespoons water

- 2 large bunch fresh cilantro, chopped

- 2 teaspoon cinnamon

- 1 teaspoon saffron

- 2 tablespoons sea salt

- 2 teaspoon paprika

- 2 teaspoon turmeric

- A dash of fresh lemon juice

Instructions

1. Rinse and dry chicken and place onto a clean plate.
2. For the marinade: In a large bowl, mix three
3. tablespoons water, the cilantro, cinnamon, saffron, salt, half the onions, garlic, cumin, ginger, paprika, and turmeric. Mix thoroughly, crush

the garlic with your fingers, and add a little water to make a paste.

4. Roll the chicken pieces into the marinade and leave for at least 25 to 30 minutes.

5. To cook, place in a casserole dish or slow cooker with the rest of the onions. Simmer on low for 6 0 minutes to

6. (While chicken is cooking excess juices will bubble up and pool around the edges of the tagine; just carefully ladle the juice out into a bowl. After the

7. chicken is cooked transfer the bowl of juices to a saucepan and cook on high, reducing the liuid for about 6 minutes -- essentially making a gravy -- and serve on top of the chicken.)

Dukan Pumpkin Brownies

Ingredients

- 1/2 cup cocoa (no sugar variety)

- 1/2 cup sweetener (i used sugar twin, brown)

- 2 tsp baking soda

- 2 tsp vanilla extract 2 fresh egg

- Dash of milk

- 2 cup oat bran

- 1 cup pumpkin

- 450 grams tofu

Instructions

1. Mix everything together, and mix well! Cook for 25
2. minutes at 46 0 degrees.
3. This makes uite a big tray, and gives us a huge
4. serving when divided by 6 .
5. It taste absolutely marvelous without icing.

Low Carb Pizza

Ingredients:

• Low carb, sugar free tomato sauce (homemade would be good)

• Vegetables (pepper, onion, mushrooms)

• Turkey Pepperoni

• 1/2 cup No Fat Cottage Cheese

• Whole cauliflower, or small bag of frozen

• 2 fresh egg, or 1/2 cup egg creations

• Random spices

Method

1. Boil or steam your Cauliflower. Then 'rice' in food processor or blender. Make sure you've tried to get as
2. much water out of it as possible.
3. Then, add spices to 'riced' cauliflower, and 2 fresh egg or fresh egg creations, and mix up.
4. Spread Cauliflower mixture into casserole dish and mash down until crust like.
5. Bake for 25 minutes at 430 degrees.
6. Pour tomato sauce on to baked 'crust' and top your pizza the way you wish.
7. I used green peppers, mushrooms, and turkey pepperon) (2% fat, zero carbs)
8. Add cottage cheese to top of pizza. Bake your pizza

9. for 30 minutes at 430 degrees.

Oat Bran Porridge

Ingredients

- 3 tablespoons of Oat Bran

- 200mls of skimmed milk

- 2 teaspoons of allowed sweetener

Instructions

1. Tip the Oat Bran into a microwaveable dish, add the
2. milk and the sweetener and mix. Microwave of full power for two minutes, stir then microwave for one
3. more minute.

4. Remove from microwave, stir well, allow to cool for a minute or two then enjoy.

Moussaka

Ingredients

- 1 lb.minced turkey or beef

- 2 onion, diced

- 2 eggplant, peeled and sliced fairly thinly

- 2 tablespoons fat-free cream cheese i used FF

fromage fraise

- 1/2 cup fat-free plain yogurt

- Good shake of nutmeg salt and pepper (to taste) Instructions

Preheat oven to 4 6 0 degrees.

- 1 can chopped tomatoes , drained

- 4 oz. mushrooms, sliced

- 1/2 cup fresh parsley

- 2 clove garlic, chopped

- 1 tblespoon dried oregano

- 1 tblespoon dried rosemary

- 2 teaspoon cinnamon

- 2 fresh egg + 2 fresh egg white

Prepare mixture one:

1. Brown mince with onion in a frying pan sprayed with frylite or similar.
2. Add aubergine, tomatoes, mushrooms, parsley, garlic, oregano, rosemary, cinnamon, salt and pepper.

3. Cook until aubergine is tender (about 25 minutes).

Prepare topping

1. Blend together the eggs, cream cheese, yogurt, nutmeg, and 1 t. of salt until smooth.
2. Place meat mixture in a casserole dish.
3. Layer mixture topping onto meat mixture
4. Sprinkle top with cinnamon.
5. Bake in oven for25-30 minutes until top is set.

Crispy Chicken Wings

MAKES 2 SERVINGS

1/2 cup low-sodium soy sauce

2 garlic clove, crushed

2 teaspoons zero-calorie sweetener suited for cooking and baking, such as Splenda, dissolved in 2 teaspoon water

4 teaspoons five-spice powder (star anise, cloves, pepper, cinnamon, fennel)

2 teaspoon peeled and chopped fresh ginger

6 chicken wings, tips cut off (see Note)

2 . In a medium dish, combine the soy sauce, garlic, sweetener, five-spice powder, and ginger.

2. Place the chicken wings in the dish and set in the refrigerator to marinate for 2 to 4 hours, turning them over once or twice.

4 . Turn the oven on to Broil, and preheat for 10 minutes.

4. Place the chicken in a roasting pan. Cook under the broiler for 4 to 10 minutes, or until the wings start to hiss and crackle. Turn the wings over and cook for an additional 4 to 10 minutes, or until golden brown.

6 . Remove the chicken from the oven and discard the skin before eating.

Chicken Broth With Mussels

Salt and freshly ground black pepper

2 pounds 4 ounces mussels

6 fresh chives, chopped

2 tablespoons chopped fresh parsley or chervil

4 pounds 6 ounces chicken wing tips

2 onions

2 shallots

2 head of garlic, cloves separated

4 stalks of celery

2 bouuet garni (make your own by tying together 6 sprigs of fresh parsley, 4 sprigs of fresh thyme, and 4 dried bay leaves)

1. Place 4 quarts of slightly salted water in a large pot and bring to a boil. Add the chicken wing tips, onions, shallots, garlic, celery, bouuet garni, and pepper to taste to the water.
2. Cover the pot and simmer for 2 hours over very low heat, taking care not to boil the broth (boiling will make the broth become cloudy).
3. Strain the cooked broth, bring to a boil, and add salt and pepper to taste.
4. Scrub and rinse the mussels several times. Discard any shells that are

open or broken and that do not close when tapped.

5. Place the mussels in a large, high-sided frying pan with a lid, and add 2 cup of water.

6. Cook over high heat until the liuid comes to a boil. Reduce the heat to a simmer, cover the pot, and cook for about 4 minutes, until the mussels open. Discard any unopened mussels.

7. Strain the mussels and save the cooking juices. Shell the mussels, but leave

8. a few unshelled in reserve to garnish the broth.

9. Divide the shelled mussels among six bowls, adding a little of the cooking juices.

10. To serve, pour the chicken broth over the mussels, sprinkle with the

chopped herbs, and garnish with the unshelled mussels. Serve immediately.

Thai Chicken Broth

2 fresh kaffir lime leaves, chopped, or 2 teaspoons grated lime zest

2 tablespoon peeled and chopped fresh ginger

Salt and freshly ground black pepper

2 chicken carcasses

2 onion, uartered

2 bunch of fresh cilantro, roughly chopped

2 fresh lemongrass stalks (white parts only), crushed

126

1. Put the chicken carcasses into a large pot and add 2 uarts of cold water. Bring to a boil, and with a ladle skim off and discard the scum that rises to the top.

2. Reduce the heat, and add the onion, cilantro, lemongrass, kaffir lime leaves or lime zest, and ginger to the pot. Cover and simmer over very low heat for 21 hours, taking care not to boil (boiling will make the broth become cloudy). Strain the broth and add salt and pepper to taste before serving.

Mustardy Chicken Kebabs

- 4 boneless, skinless chicken breasts
- 2 low-sodium chicken bouillon cube
- 2 tablespoons Dijon mustard
- 2 teaspoon fresh lemon juice
- 2   garlic clove, chopped 2   teaspoon cornstarch
- 1/2 cup cold fat-free milk

1. Cut the chicken breasts into 2 -inch chunks and put them in a large nonreactive bowl.
2. In a medium bowl, dissolve the bouillon cube in 2 cup of hot water.
3. Add the mustard, lemon juice, and garlic. Pour three-quarters of this marinade over the chicken, mix thoroughly, cover, and refrigerate for 2 hours.
4. Preheat oven to 450°F.
5. Thread the chicken chunks onto skewers (see Note) and place on a rack over a rimmed baking sheet. Roast them for about 8 minutes, or until just cooked through.
6. In a small saucepan, blend the cornstarch with the cold milk and add the remaining quarter of the marinade. Gently simmer the mixture

over medium heat, stirring often, for 10 minutes, or until the sauce thickens. Serve alongside the kebabs.

7. Note: You will need 8 wooden or metal skewers for this recipe. If you are using wooden skewers, soak them in water for at least 45 minutes before using them so they won't burn.

Spicy Chicken Kebabs

2 teaspoon peeled and grated fresh ginger

2 garlic clove, crushed

2 pounds 4 ounces boneless, skinless chicken breasts, cut into 2 -inch cubes

2 cup fat-free plain Greek-style yogurt

2 teaspoon chili powder

2 teaspoon ground turmeric

2 teaspoon ground cumin

2 teaspoon ground coriander

1. In a medium bowl, combine the yogurt, chili, turmeric, cumin, coriander, ginger, and garlic.
2. Thread the chicken pieces onto skewers and place in a dish big enough for the skewers to lie flat.
3. Cover the chicken with the marinade and place in the refrigerator, covered, for several hours or overnight.
4. When the chicken has marinated, heat up the barbecue or turn the oven on to Broil, and preheat for 10 minutes.
5. Place the kebabs under the broiler or on the barbecue and cook until the meat is browned and tender, about 8 minutes.

Herb-Stuffed Chicken Legs

25 fresh chives, finely chopped

Salt and freshly ground black pepper

2 chicken legs with thighs attached, skin removed

⅓ cup fat-free plain Greek-style yogurt

2 shallot, chopped

2 tablespoon chopped fresh parsley

1. Preheat oven to 4 8 6 °F.
2. In a medium bowl, combine the yogurt, shallot, parsley, and chives. Season with salt and pepper to taste.
3. Using a sharp, pointed knife, make an incision into the thickest part of each chicken thigh, about 5 inches long and 2 inch deep.
4. Push the yogurt mixture into the slits and coat the chicken thighs with the rest of the mixture.
5. Cut out two 8 × 8-inch sheets of aluminum foil and place a chicken thigh in the center of each piece, closing the foil to form a parcel.
6. Put a little water in the bottom of a small baking dish and place the parcels in it.
7. Bake in the oven for 45 minutes.

Tandoori Chicken

6 boneless, skinless chicken breasts

4 garlic cloves, crushed

2 teaspoons peeled and very finely chopped fresh ginger

2 fresh green chili peppers, very finely chopped

2 cup fat-free plain Greek-style yogurt

2 teaspoons tandoori masala spice mix

Juice of 2 fresh lemon

Salt and freshly ground black pepper

1. Put each chicken breast on a sheet of plastic wrap and beat with a rolling pin until 1/2 inch thick.
2. In a medium nonreactive bowl, mix together the garlic, ginger, chilies, yogurt, tandoori masala, and fresh lemon juice until thoroughly combined. Add salt and pepper to taste.
3. Make several ⅛-inch-deep incisions into each chicken breast. Place the chicken in a glass baking dish and thoroughly coat with the yogurt mixture. Cover and refrigerate overnight.
4. The following day, preheat the oven to 400°F.
5. Cook the chicken for 10 minutes, then turn the oven temperature up to

Broil and cook for an additional 2 minutes, or until brown.

Barbecued Curry Chicken

4 boneless, skinless chicken breasts

2 cup fat-free plain Greek-style yogurt

2 tablespoon curry powder

Salt and freshly ground black pepper

Put each chicken breast on a sheet of plastic wrap and beat with a rolling pin until 1/2 inch thick.

In a small bowl, mix together the yogurt and curry powder, and add salt and pepper to taste.

Place the chicken in a glass baking dish and thoroughly coat with the yogurt mixture. Cover with plastic wrap and allow the chicken to marinate for 2 hours in the refrigerator.

When the chicken has marinated, heat up the barbecue or turn the oven on to Broil and preheat for 10 minutes.

Barbecue or broil the chicken pieces for 10 minutes, turning once.

Lemongrass Chicken

⅛ teaspoon vegetable oil

4 pounds 6 ounces boneless, skinless chicken breasts, cut into ¼-inch strips

2 small onions, finely chopped

4 fresh lemongrass stalks, white parts only, finely chopped

A pinch of chili powder

2 tablespoons nuoc mam (Vietnamese fish sauce)

2 tablespoons low-sodium soy sauce

2 tablespoons zero-calorie sweetener suited for cooking and baking, such as Splenda

1. Salt and freshly ground black pepper
2. Heat a large, heavy-bottomed skillet over medium heat. Add the oil and wipe out any excess with a paper towel.
3. Add the chicken and cook, stirring often, until brown.
4. Add the onions, lemongrass, chili powder, nuoc mam, soy sauce, sweetener, and salt and pepper to taste.
5. Lower the heat, cover the pan, and cook for 30 minutes.

145

Lightning Source UK Ltd.
Milton Keynes UK
UKHW022023240123
415919UK00020B/215

9 781990 207785